Herbert Anthem, Ph.D.

I0438369

Coping with Hand & Arm Pain:

Dueling Medical Reports and the Single Payer Health Care Option

© 2011 Herbert Anthem, Ph.D.

Herbert Anthem, Ph.D.

First Paperback Edition 2011

Cataloging Information:
Anthem, Herbert.
     Coping with Hand & Arm Pain: Dueling Medical Reports
     and the Single Payer Health Care Option
        p. cm.
    ISBN-10: 1460985176   ISBN-13: 978-1460985175
        1. National health care. 2. Hand injury. 3. Personal
     injury litigation process in the United States. 4. Self
     care. 5. Professional development. 6. Memoir.
R151.A   362.11 A

herbertanthem@dr.com
Also Available in Large Print Edition:
ISBN-13: 978-1461028291

Distribution of this title is through
Ingram/LSI and Baker & Taylor.

Also available for purchase online.

Preface

A case study is presented in this volume as a personal memoir. The author is not a licensed physician, nor a health care provider of any kind. The case study is from the experience of having a significant injury and seeking treatment and cure over a fifteen year period within four states in the United States. Many of the discoveries made through experience were quite surprising and encompass learning how medical science actually functions in the United States, the role of exploring herbal remedies, and the roles of law, litigation, and social safety nets.

The experiences were further explored through research, including interviews with other injured people, disabled homeless people, and interviews with numerous health care providers.

An unexpected discovery was why a single payer health care system cannot work in the United States *under the current laws in the various states and federal court system*. The problem is one that trial lawyers and the physicians who write medical reports for them already know but do not share with the general public.

Along the way, finding a personal cure is discussed.

Herbert Anthem, Ph.D.

Notes:

Herbert Anthem, Ph.D.

Table of Contents

Herbert Anthem, Ph.D.

Notes:

Herbert Anthem, Ph.D.

Coping with

Hand & Arm

Pain

Herbert Anthem, Ph.D.

Notes:

Herbert Anthem, Ph.D.

1. Onset and Diagnosis

Perhaps you or someone in your family or one of your friends or co-workers or neighbors has developed hand, wrist, and/or forearm pain. That certainly can be a life changing experience! What you thought you knew about how American culture works rapidly proves to be untrue. Safety nets break — fast — and formerly well off individuals can rapidly find themselves in unexpected stress as the result of any injury, especially repetitive motion injuries sustained on the job. The general public expects that either Workers Compensation, Unemployment Insurance, Social Security, Medicare, or Medicaid will break their fall and prevent their complete impoverishment. However, there are only three really protective resources: private long care insurance, family wealth, or national health care.

Medical science and herb shops did not alleviate my hand, wrist, and forearm pain. In fact, the *carpel tunnel* portion of my repetitive motion injury got so bad that the nerve hurt all up my arm, through the neck segment of the spine, and up through the right side of my face — through the teeth and the right eye. There was also *de Quervain's tenosynovitis, bracheitis, neural spasm,* and *radial nerve neuritis.* The right hand, wrist, and forearm up to the elbow were in bad shape, and the left arm rapidly developed *carpel tunnel* and *bracheitis* as that arm tried to carry the whole workload. My pain was not eliminated by prescription medication, nor braces, nor chiropractic, nor physical therapy — though all of those did help at least to some extent. My pain was eliminated by a product I bought and continue to buy in dollar stores for $1.

In fact, it took six years to find any prescription medication that reduced the *chronic pain* in my right hand, wrist, and forearm below my *pain threshold.* Figuratively, I had been climbing the walls in pain for six years. Typically, I would show up in hospital emergency rooms, wrap my arm from the elbow down in wet paper towels, and pace the floor until a physician would write either *Percocet, Toradol,* or *Ketorolac* prescription for temporary relief. Sometimes the prescription was for *Tylenol 3,* the kind with *codeine.*

I had to drive 100 miles to get home on the first, hospital dispensed prescription for *Percocet.* Fortunately, I never took the entire dosage at once, since my individual tolerance for that compound proved to be very low. It would have become my drug of choice except that I, personally, felt like a balloon flying around on a long string in a brisk wind when I took that medication. If I had had no responsibilities, it would have been a different matter, and I might have simply enjoyed the balloon ride.

The other two prescriptions I was typically given were for intense, post surgery pain and were not for routine maintenance of an *inflammatory condition*. *Tylenol 3* (with *codeine*) was prescribed and worked for me, but again, I was told that is for crisis level pain, not for maintenance medication.

Physicians got around to telling me that what I had was an *inflammatory condition* of the right arm. Later, physicians termed it an *inflammatory disease* of the right arm, since it didn't go away as they had hoped. However, I never knew what to believe, since the first hand specialist I consulted informed me that I had:

> *rheumatism; get use to it. Professors don't work hard enough to sustain repetitive motion injuries to their hands. You're just getting old.*

He was wrong. The other physicians I consulted

agreed that I did not have *rheumatism*, nor *arthritis*.

I had to go out of state during the second year of my arm condition in order to find really good care — and I lived in a modern, industrialized state as it was.

The most effective brace I was prescribed during the first five years immobilized my right arm in thick plastic from the palm to half way between the elbow and shoulder. Wisely, that hand specialist informed me that all of the major structures from the wrist to the elbow were connected at each end. He said that a brace that merely immobilized the wrist could never be expected to do the job. The elbow had to be immobilized, too. He told me that information after others had prescribed short braces, and those had failed to do the job. My right arm condition had worsened beyond the assistance of the short braces despite two *corticosteroid* injections in less than a year.

You can imagine how people reacted to seeing my right arm in a heavy plastic brace from the palm to five inches above the elbow! A person can't drive in such a brace, nor cook, nor dress, nor groom, etc., etc. People asked me if I had broken my arm. Many thought the fancy brace was a new treatment for a broken bone.

One hostile physician actually told me not to tell

anyone that I had wrist pain, lest I be thought to masturbate. I suppose that social threat intimidates many single and married alike, men and women alike. But it makes just as much sense to tell a person that he or she has developed wrist pain as the result of too much heterosexual sex. What the heck should we think of the theory of evolution, if men have not evolved to use their wrists to support themselves during sex or if women have not developed wrists strong enough to caress a man to climax? Wrists have had that repetitive work to sustain for thousands of years, if not for millennia.

I've never heard of anyone going around saying that their wrists hurt because they had too active a sex life. It is not sex that has changed all that much; it is repetitive work conditions on the jobs during the post-industrial age that the hands, wrists, and forearms can't keep up with and repetitive sports such as tennis and handball. Prior to the post-industrial age, *de Quervains* was a washerwoman's injury rather than one sustained by physicians, dentists, and editors as it is now.

Some physicians claim that the smaller hand structures of women are more prone to injury than the larger hand structures of men. Some physicians claim that women don't do work that is demanding enough to cause hand or wrist injuries. If so, why is it that we see so many grocery clerks wearing wrist braces? Who is going to suggest with any chance of success that for some reason grocery store clerks masturbate more than the general public?

For six years, I tried at least six different *hand specialists* in four states, a *neurologist*, three *chiropractors*, and had sessions with several *physical therapists*. Lots of things helped a little for a short while. *Corticosteroid* injections felt good for three weeks at a time. *Chiropractic* sessions helped for three days at a time. Heat helped. Cold helped. Nothing worked for the long term. I was taken off work duty for one academic term, and my hand, wrist, and forearm pain did not go away.

Then six years after the onset of the cruel level of pain, a medical resident thought of *gabapentin*. That took away 80% of my pain in twenty minutes. I called my relatives immediately and reported the news that there was a drug that worked for me that I would probably need for the rest of my life. At the time, it was a wonderful relief. I was wrong.

I cannot recommend *gabapentin* for others, of course, since I am not a medical doctor and since a number of people I interviewed reported that they personally found that it upsets their stomach. Pharmacists can give you details on that, so can websites. (Checking the pill books at your public library reference section can assist you in researching side effects.) However, at the time, I was very grateful for that prescription. I encourage anyone with chronic pain to discuss *gabapentin* with their own physician(s). The problem I have is that my *pain threshold* is so very high that once my hand and wrist pain started, it was already almost too late.

Physicians I interviewed agreed that *gabapentin* was invented for *epileptics* as an *anti-spasmodic*. *Epileptics* who had *chronic pain* reported reduction in their *chronic pain*, and there were attempts to separate the *anti-spasmodic* qualities from the pain reducing qualities, but those efforts did not work. Instead, *gabapentin* became cross licensed by the FDA for both *epilepsy* and for *chronic pain*.

Physicians I interviewed also reported that *gabapentin* is also used as a *mood stabilizer*, so there are several medical conditions for which licensed physicians prescribe *gabapentin*. Physicians pick according to their professional judgment. You can inquire of your licensed physician for his or her advice concerning the appropriateness of this medication, if you have a *chronic pain* condition. I have found physicians well informed concerning this medication. Some medications work well on acute (new) pain; some work on chronic; some work on both. Your physicians and your pharmacists can tell you which to try for your ailment with the greatest likelihood of success.

I discovered that I could not take the *gabapentin* capsules long term at the strengths that the physicians wanted me to take. The *mood stabilizer* aspect would kick in and take away my ability to appreciate the visual beauty of nature — a delight upon which I rely. My physicians adjusted the dosage downward, and we found a maintenance level. I was told that dosages decline with age as a result of more mature people being able to metabolize *gabapentin* more efficiently than do young people.

Since ejaculation and orgasm and birth delivery contractions and heart beats are spasmodic responses of the body, I gave some thought to that. As decades pass, perhaps there will be greater success in separating out the *anti-spasmodic*, *chronic pain* alleviation, and mood stabilizing chemistry of *gabapentin* into three separate and distinct formulations. None of my physicians said any word about the *anti-spasmodic* aspect with regard to ejaculation/orgasm or birth delivery contractions or heart beats, but patients are another matter. They openly discuss these matters with each other.

At the point *gabapentin* was prescribed to me for the first time, six years into my *inflammatory condition*, I believed we had reached the most effective treatment that medical science could find. By the ten year marker, hundreds of thousands of dollars in medical care had been racked up in efforts to treat and cure my conditions.

2. *Seeking Alternatives*

The first summer of my *de Quervain's tenosynovitis*, which proved to be the major diagnosis, a friend of mine suggested that I try *Essiac*, or *Cassie's Tea*. This is a compound of Ojibwa, Native Canadian, medicine used by a nurse by the name of Cassie in Canada against cancer for some 40 years. The *immune system booster* is said to be the ingredient *sheep sorrel*, a thin leafed lettuce that grows wild in New York State and elsewhere in North America. My helpful friend hoped that *sheep sorrel* and the three other herbs could fight off whatever I had in my right arm. However, what I had were not germs or cancers. This friend was effective in turning my attention to an exploration of herbal options beginning in the first year of my difficulty.

A relative of mine gave me one of those so called coffee table herb books for my birthday. I proceeded to put my education in scientific method to work and bought a variety of herbs plus 16 small Mason jars — the kind used for home canning. I put each herb that I bought into one of the canning jars, labeled each, and set out to conduct in formal, at home clincial trials on myself only to see if any of the herbs worked for me. What I learned is that because human metabolism is complex, different things work best for different people. Many of the herbs I tried did nothing for me that I thought was worth buying them again.

A couple of the herbs that I bought at the local herb store were interesting enough that I kept using them for some time but then stopped, since I had to eat them or drink their teas more and more to get the desired reaction. That did not seem to be a winning game as far as I was concerned.

A few of them, however, I kept up for a number of years. *Sheep sorrel* I still keep in the refrigerator. For many years, I put a pinch of *sheep sorrel* in a water bottle at the start of the day every day, and it seemed to resist my inclination towards *bronchitis*. Then I began boiling it up in a winter tea that I did not consume from October to April.

None of those herbs seemed to improve my arm conditions. I had only known about bacterial and viral infections; I had not known the characteristic of biological inflammations.

Here are some things I learned along the way to finding what did work:

One of the key problems with repetitive motion injuries to the fingers, thumb, palm, wrist, forearm, and elbow is that with excessive use of these tendons, the body pumps fluid inside the *tendon sheath*. The increase of fluid inside the tendon sheath causes swelling. In fact, my right forearm was actually measured to be ½″ larger than my left forearm in circumference during the height of pain. (This was despite my right side, in general, being physically smaller than my left side.) The swelling produced by the increased fluid is perceived by the nerves as pressure and reported to the brain as pain. Physicians and physical therapists explain this and have diagrams displaying this in detail in some of their offices.

As soon as finger, thumb, palm, wrist, forearm, elbow, upper arm, and/or shoulder pain is perceived, a person needs to consult a licensed physician. Waiting can cause more serious problems to develop due to aggravation of the fibers. A person's entire lifestyle can be at stake: relationships, property, career, and personal identity.

Hand specialists, specifically, come from two different branches of medicine according to physicians I have interviewed. Some begin as bone specialists — *orthopedists.* Some begin as skin specialists — *plastic surgeons.* Both *orthopedists* and *plastic surgeons* learn the other specialty over time as they practice medicine. So, when patients consult a *hand specialist,* the patient can ask the physician whether he or she began as an *orthopedist* or as a *plastic surgeon.*

Just as you need to know that you can communicate with your physicians, your physicians need to know that they can communicate with you. If you demonstrate to them that you can comprehend their explanations, they will tend to give fuller explanations. We can't expect physicians to gage our level of understanding accurately, if we do not communicate with them openly. As I learned to tell them what I already knew, they tended to provide additional details, adding to my information and my ability to increase in self care. Sometimes just asking a hand specialist whether he or she came from *orthopedics* or *plastic surgery* opened up the communications channels to more detailed explanations. That one question signaled a level of prior coaching from previous physicians.

Hand specialists tend to be called on to repair and reconstruct digits, hands, arms, toes, feet, and/or ankles that have gotten crushed or severed. They really do masterful work that saves the quality of life for many patients.

The first lines of defense that they recommended to me were wearing a brace at night and taking an over the counter *anti-inflammatory*. Many people go buy an off the rack brace and an over the counter *anti-inflammatory* without consulting a licensed physician. I believe that people make a mistake when they do not immediately consult a physician. I believe it is important to consult a physician immediately even if that strains the budget. It is also useful to follow up immediately by getting a second opinion.

This is because life in contemporary America is highly dependent upon having the use of hands. People cannot even manage application for their safety net benefits, if they do not have use of their hands. Every American is assumed to have some minimal level of paper processing, form processing ability. If people neglect their hand health, they can lose their paper processing, their form processing ability. Hand injuries can impact a person's entire quality of life.

Orthopedists can tend to do a heavy practice in hip and knee replacements, since their specialty is founded on a profound understanding of the bones and how the bones function. While plastic surgeons learn the body from the skin in, orthopedists learn the body from the bones out. Both fields are capable of full mastery, whether they begin from the outside and go inward or whether they begin with the inside and go outward.

A variety of hand, wrist, and forearm injuries exist. Faculty members who tend to do a large volume of grading/paper marking might develop *trigger finger*. High school faculty can develop this. One of the treatments for *trigger finger* is surgery. Guitarists might develop a particular thumb condition from holding the guitar pick and strumming with frequency and duration. Arthritis and rheumatism do cause problems with fingers and with joints. *De Quervain's tenosynovitis* is a condition in the tendon that attaches the base of the thumb diagonally to the outer side of the elbow. People — such as dentists, surgeons, and line editors — who use a fine implement might develop this condition. Dentists and surgeons tend to cut back their practice schedules as soon as *de Quervain's tenosynovitis* symptoms appear, since these medical practitioners tend to be aware of the seriousness of the threat that the condition poses to their careers. In the time before automatic washing machines, this condition use to be contracted by washerwomen.

Bracheitis used to be known as *tennis elbow*. However, it can occur along with *de Quervain's tenosynovitis* in fine implement use when both the thumb and index finger are stressed. The term *bracheitis* now acknowledges that playing tennis is not the only cause of forearm pain. The condition has also been termed *brachial radial tendonitis*. The terms used by health care professionals can change over time in some specialties, so sometimes you might come to find your condition labeled differently than it was in the past.

Physical sites of hand, wrist, and arm pains include in the fingers, in the webbing between the thumb and palm, below the base of the thumb, at the front side of the elbow and elsewhere. The reason why braces tend to provide some assistance is that some people tend to sleep with their wrists bent, which does not allow free circulation of blood

through the wrist, hand, thumb, and fingers overnight.
Reduced circulation can have some impact on the ability of
the body to heal overnight from daily use. Wearing a brace
prevents the individual from folding his or her wrist over
and sleeping on it overnight. Compressing the *arteries and
the veins* in that position can reduce the flow of circulation
and the delivery of nutrients to fibers that are trying to heal.

Anti-inflammatories work by means of decreasing the
pressure from the build-up of water, so that the body does
not report excessive pressure as pain. Also, my physicians
reported that the body needs all of the B vitamins in order
to heal. I was repeatedly told to take an over the counter, *B
complex* vitamin pill daily. Those B vitamins need to be
consumed *and* circulated in order to reach the desired
destinations.

The two middle fingers and the little finger of my right
hand have never been a problem except that when the
inflammatory condition is extreme, my right hand will
freeze up. My physicians have called this immobility *neural
spasm. Neural spasms* look peculiar, but I don't experience
neural spasm as pain, and I find that distraction works the
best to stop it. During the *spasm*, orders from the brain to
the hand do not seem to get through the nervous system

from one point to the other. If I will concentrate on something else entirely, some casual thought to perform some casual gesture seems to get through after a while, and the hand becomes flexible again.

The pain that I had from the inside palm to the inside of the elbow was a symptom that my physicians called *radial nerve neuritis*. This reduced my grip strength. My pinch strength was reduced to two pounds.

The reason why I mention these terms to you is so that you will be able to communicate with your physicians better. You can ask which of these terms apply in your own personal circumstances. Your medical team may teach you entirely different terms to apply to yourself and their treatment of you. That would be a good outcome.

Comfrey was among the herbs that my friend drew my attention to during that first summer when my pain symptoms appeared. For the initial six years of my ailment, *comfrey* was the only substance that seemed to make a lasting difference. *Comfrey* is said to work on the same parts of the body that a host ovum cell controls during genetic engineering experiments. These structures, if I recall correctly, are skin, bone, and sinew — *not* organ genetics.

Comfrey is traditionally said to stimulate the body to heal itself—but not the organs.

Again, what I read during research in herb books did not tell me anything about doses. By trial and error, I discovered that my body accepted *comfrey* best as a lotion. I would put about 1/3 cup of dry comfrey into a 4 or 8 ounce bottle of olive oil and let it sit for at least a week. When I remembered to do so, I would shake up the bottle. The longer the *comfrey* steeped in the olive oil, the better the lotion seemed to become.

Comfrey gives the olive oil a green hue. Since the green tint can come off onto clothing, I would lather my right hand and forearm in the lotion, cover with paper toweling, and wear clothing that did not matter. During the first 3 to 4 days, this seemed to have no effect. On about the 4th day, I began to feel some lessening of the pain.

I used the *comfrey* for over six years. I did not discontinue it when I began taking *gabapentin capsules*. I did discontinue the *comfrey* once my arm pain subsided below threshold on a day to day basis. I did not require all of the pain to go away. I required that the pain stay below my personal tolerance threshold.

There was one very interesting incident with the *comfrey*. I tried it as a tea, and that was too strong for me. I did not like the side effects. I also would put a heaping tablespoon quantity in the palm of my hand and toss the *comfrey* into a tub of warm to hot water and soak in it as a therapeutic soak. There was one day when I got into the tub with bruises on both my calves from gardening. When I got into the tub, I noticed the bruises and was annoyed, since as it happened, my calves were going to be on public display that summer evening. To my complete amazement, when I got out of the tub after a half hour soak in the *comfrey* saturated water — the bruises had vanished! This proved to me to my satisfaction that my skin, at least, responded well to the herb *comfrey*.

But *comfrey* is not the mystery herb that cured my right arm.

3. *Physical Therapies*

Mechanical treatments of various sorts were tried in the efforts of my physicians and physical therapists to heal my injured right arm. Some of these treatments were combined with exercises. Both hot compresses and cold compresses felt good. Despite everyone's best efforts, I occasionally flunked my *physical therapy* sessions .

During the initial treatment, a bath sheet was saturated with water and frozen by the physical therapist. My right arm was then wrapped up in that frozen towel for 20 minutes prior to my being taught a series of hand exercises to maintain flexibility and to avoid *fibroid tumors*. The icing treatment took 20 very painful minutes. The hand exercises took five minutes. I did not go back for a second session. The icing of my forearm and hand was too painful!

The finger exercises were a series of stretches, lifts, and curls. All of the digits were to be stretched out widely five times and relaxed five times. Each of the digits was to be lifted off the surface of a table one at a time while the palm remained in contact with the table surface. That was to be repeated five times. All of the fingers were to be curled in toward the palm five times and relaxes five times. My physicians insisted that I do the curls with the thumb ending up outside the fingers rather than inside of them in the curl, since the pressure was too great on my thumb inside of the curl. Thus, I was given three exercises to repeat five times off and on throughout the day and night – just to retain tone and flexibility. Initially, I did these very rarely because the exercises were too painful to do. It was hard enough trying to get by with just routine, daily, self care.

Other injured people reported to me that they were set to kneading sand or unpopped popcorn that filled basins for wrist conditions that differed from mine.

One thing that I have never understood is why physical therapy massage worked although I experienced pain when even a baby touched my right arm. I am prepared to believe that massage worked for *psychosomatic* reasons. If that is not the reason, then it might be that accidentally being poked by a baby startled me while the touch of the physical therapist was expected and thus not so much of a jolt.

I was taught ways of placing my palms open on a wall and leaning into the wall to improve muscle tone through tension. That exercise felt good. Nothing touched my arms in that exercise, yet the muscles got a workout.

It is highly valuable to have a series of *physical therapy* each time a physician offers that and even to go to different *physical therapists*. They do have different routines that they prefer, and the routines that they prefer change over time. All insurances seem to have limits to the number of *physical therapy* visits, but sometimes physicians can write letters to the insurance to justify additional sessions, as with *chiropractic*.

Physical therapists told me that I had to avoid using ice packs for longer than 20 minutes at a time, since icing for longer than that could cause damage my tissues. They also told me that there are two simple, homemade ice packs. One is to use a bag of frozen peas or frozen corn after loosening the vegetables inside the plastic bag. I never did that because I knew that the touch of the solid surface on my skin would be painful. I was also told that a plastic baggie filled with 50% water and 50% rubbing alcohol would freeze up into a slush that would work as an ice pack. I did try that once, but the pressure would be painful against my skin.

What I was able to use was cold or hot water. Hydrotherapy did work for me. Unfortunately, showering became a challenge because the water pressure hurt my skin. However, hydrotherapy did work for me. For almost two years I kept a pool/health club membership in order to use the hot tubs. Immersing my arms in hot tubs and in swimming pools was the kind of hydrotherapy my injuries responded to in addition to bathtub soaking.

When a chiropractor used a sonic wand inside a bucket of water with my arm in it, that made my arm feel better, also. Of course, I realize that the effect might have been from soaking my arm in the cold water. When I got a spa membership and soaked frequently in a hot tub, that seemed to improve the circulation in my arm and reduce the pain. I continue to believe that the hot tub treatment was useful. It was time consuming. I would go to the spa and go into the hot tub for up to the maximum 15 minutes allowed, get out, wait, and then repeat the treatment through an entire day, several days a week—sometimes every day.

During the summer, soaking in a cool pool made my swollen arms feel better. During the winter, soaking in the hot tub made my chilled arms fell better. My arms in general were more painful during weather over 70 degrees Fahrenheit. An *anesthesiologist* who was a *pain specialist* explained to me that icy weather during the winter functions as a natural anesthetic, reducing the pain of my *inflammatory condition*. Individuals I have interviewed who have *arthritic conditions* reported that their pain lessens during the heat of summer. Medical specialists manage the two kinds of conditions differently, and it is important to be under the supervision of the appropriate medical specialists.

Each of the prescribed hand/wrist/arm braces that I was prescribed was wonderful in its own way. There were plastic ones molded specifically to my arms. We began with right forearm ones and progressed into adding left forearm ones. Each of these began at the palm.

There were cloth braces that were reinforced with metal or stiff plastic spines. The first two of these were basically soft, padded cylinders with thumb holes. The right hand one had a right hand thumb hole; the left one had a left thumb hole. These first two cloth braces were for use while driving. I have always worn my braces with the thumbs tucked in, since my thumbs are the most significant problem. The plastic splints have thumb sprockets specifically to immobilize the thumb.

Physicians told me to always insist on a *cocked wrist splint*. These have the palm tilted back slightly at an angle. This keeps the inside *tendons* tensed and the outside tendons flexed in a relaxed posture.

Just imagine my going out in public with both hands, wrists, and forearms splinted inside plastic braces. Anytime I had to interact with educated people, they tended to become shocked and traumatized just by seeing both arms splinted up. People would demand, 'You are getting better, right?' They tended to ask this while poking my upper arm with a jabbing finger. I tended to yelp or hit the ceiling, depending on the day.

If I did not wear my braces, people tended to say, 'You don't look disabled.'

Even though I was forbidden from wearing my braces 24 hours a day, if I did not wear them when I was in public, the public seemed unable to comprehend that I was disabled. The public does not seem to understand mechanical problems with the body unless appliances are required: braces, canes, wheelchairs, etc. The public also does not seem to understand that while certain ailments require resting the body part in a brace, the body part can also require resting from the brace.

An injured tendon does not heal in the identical manner as an injured bone, since tendons break in ways that differ from the ways in which bones break. Tendons swell from inflammations; bones crack, splinter, or break apart. While bracing an inflamed hand/wrist/arm to immobilize it is done for only part of a 24 hour period, casts for broken bones sometimes remain on continuously for weeks/months. Removing a brace from an inflamed hand/wrist/arm does not mean the body part is well; it means that the individual has been instructed to do so by his/her physician.

In fact, I begged my physicians to brace my right fingers, hand, wrist, and arm more; I was told they would not and could not, since they knew of patients who had developed fibroid tumors from such measures. If casting inflamed hands, wrists, and arms worked, physicians would put them in the kinds of casts broken bones require to heal properly. The conditions are very different and are braced differently.

The *chiropractors* hooked me up to tingling electrodes. Two physicians performed *nerve tests*, which they warned me about. Apparently, many patients experience *nerve testing* as being highly painful. I reported to both physicians that *nerve testing* was some of the most soothing *physical therapy* I had experienced.

The slight electrical current that was sent through my right arm nerves made those raw and painful nerves feel better. If I could have had a weekly treatment, I would have reported back again and again until the effect changed. My experience was as though my stinging nerves were massaged inside my body by the electrical current used in the testing.

All of the health providers repeatedly inquired about *numbness* or *tingling* in my fingers. Each exam included *range of motion testing*. During testing for *range of motion*, I was told to lift my arms in a variety of ways and move them around in a variety of ways. Since my shoulders were not the problem, I could lift and move my arms. Opening a letter or writing were impossible. Coordinating my two hands to do something together was impossible. For example, I became unable to wear shoes that had tied laces.

I almost never experienced any *numbness* or *tingling*

and always had full *range of motion*. Everything worked physically. The fingers, thumb, and wrist on the right side hurt too much to be used. Despite that, the physicians kept telling me I had to keep my fingers in use in order to avoid *fibroid tumors*. I have not to date gotten any.

I was given a *paraffin wax*, hand appliance (that can also be used for candle dipping). What I learned from this hand spa was to make certain to allow the wax to cool sufficiently before dipping either hand/wrist into the wax. Although the wax melting temperature is set very low to avoid combustion of the *paraffin*, the melted wax temperature is still too hot for the skin. After the wax has melted, turn the heating element off and allow the wax to re-cool before dipping the hands in. There is a cool down temperature at which the heat will not redden the skin and yet the wax is still liquid. That is what is sought.

Also, I discovered by trial and error that the thing for me to do was to re-dip and re-dip both of my hand/wrists into the wax until an eighth to ¼″ covering of wax built up. Then, my hands would be completely immobilized for about a half hour while the wax cooled off. This provided deep heat treatment and a half hour of complete immobility for both hands to rest completely.   None of the braces did that. Paraffin wax treatment has been especially beneficial in the winter chill.

Those with *arthritis* and those with *inflammatory conditions* experience winter and summer differently. Cold is both a natural *anesthetic* and a natural *anti-inflammatory* that reduces the pain of *inflammatory conditions* during cold weather and inside air conditioned spaces. Even people I have met who report *arthritis* and use the paraffin wax appliance have told me they have increased pain from their condition during cold weather and reduced pain during the hot season. Those with *inflammatory conditions* report the opposite.

The best my arms get any year happens during the coldest months of each winter. Not only do I go outdoors a lot as a matter of habit, I also keep the heat closer to 65 indoors during the winter months. During the summer, I don't keep my air conditioning any lower than 80-85 when at home.

In fact, when the outdoor temperature goes into the 80s, the 90s, and to 100 during the hot season, I have felt the increments in increased pain. My pain threshold is so high that the *inflammatory response* confuses and disorients me before I feel any pain. My vision is reduced before I feel any pain.

The first time I noticed the blurred vision was when I glanced at billboard lettering while driving. It was very bewildering to look at a huge billboard and not be able to read what it said! I could see the parts of the letters that went up and those which went down, but the middles were all blurred together as the result of the chemicals my *inflammatory condition* was causing to circulate through me. We do not get told in advance to monitor our vision for *inflammatory disease* resulting from hand/wrist/forearm injuries. No physician or pharmacist has ever identified to me the exact chemicals that inflammatory disease releases into the body.

Of course, my adrenalin was high for a long time as a result of my anxiety over my medical condition. One of my physicians explained adrenal failure to me and ordered me to practice relaxation techniques to quiet the adrenals.

I learned that I would not be able to live in a region that did not have a cold winter. Living where it was warm all of the year would be physically miserable to my arms. The mechanical action of cold and hot is something I did not at all expect.

Herbert Anthem, Ph.D.

I asked several of my physicians why being in a hot tub reduced the pain in my arms and using the heated *paraffin wax* worked and why cold weather worked and small electrical currents and the other diverse treatments. I was told that at the very least the *neural pathways* get flooded, so that pain signals do not get through along the *nerves*. This was explained by describing the *neural pathway* as a door. Blocking the door up does not allow anything else to get through the door. That explains massage working, electrical stimulation working, the hot tub working, and the paraffin wax hand spa working. Cold, however, causes the fluids to contract, reducing the internal pressure that is felt as pain.

4. *The Long Haul*

As my injury went into eight and ten years, we finally arrived at some maintenance level of treatment for my arms. The left one developed *carpel tunnel* and *brachiates* over the years of having to do all the daily tasks fairly much by itself. That is called collateral injury. When I was hospitalized, one physician told me that he was going to treat both my arms just as though they were the arms of a baseball pitcher. That physician administered 12 *corticosteroid injections* within two to three months. Five injections went into my left arm, and the seven remaining injections went into my right arm.

The 12 injections were distributed such that more of the injected material went into the wrists than the front of the elbow. These were the areas where the *tendons* attached between the wrists at the thumbs and elbow and the wrists at the index finger and elbow. The first series of injections put two in my right wrist below the thumb and two in my upper forearm near the elbow at the other end of the same tendon. In my left arm, I got two injections that same day in my wrist below my left thumb and one at the opposite end of that tendon near the elbow.

I had reported to that physician that corticosteroid injections always worked for me but that they wore off after about three weeks. He had me come back after about two months. He then gave my arms an additional two injections in my wrist at the base of my right thumb and a single injection in each of the other three locations that he had previously injected. That made a tremendous and lasting difference. That physician told me that his rationale was that everything else had been tried and had failed to accomplish a cure.

He was the first physician I met who had even considered that a university professor could conceivably use his or her arms as much as a baseball pitcher does.

I was eventually given a *pain specialist* consultation, and he prescribed *lidocaine* patches. Accidentally, I touched the edge of one once to an earthworm, and the earthworm stopped moving. I have always hoped that it was only temporarily stunned. However, that gave me some additional respect for the *lidocaine* even though I did not experience a numbing sensation from it. The skin retained a sense of touch while the pain was reduced. *Pain specialists* tend to come from *anesthesiology.*

Physicians tried me on NSAIDs over the years. We tried *Tramadol, Celecoxib, Valdecoxib,* and *Diclofenac.* At one point I asked why I was not tried on all of the NSAIDs. I was told, 'You don't want to try the others.' By that I have always assumed that the others are addictive substances, but I am uncertain.

I learned to read the prescription details in books in the reserve sections of our local libraries. Those, by the way, can be fascinating in the amount of information they provide.

One herb and prescription interaction resulted in my blood pressure being measured at 200. Ironically, when I was finally granted disability status, the initiation date was the series of hospitalizations I had as a result of collapsing from high blood pressure that resulted from the drug reaction with an herb I had started taking for heart palpitations that were perhaps brought on by anxiety. It took a while to identify the interaction.

I stopped taking the herb that was interacting with the new prescription. Initially, I was not asked if I used any herbs.

Herbert Anthem, Ph.D.

The *internist* I acquired has known for many years where to check on the internet to monitor for the latest reports of herbs interacting with prescription medicine. If I decide I want to try an over the counter herb, I now ask my *internist* first, and he checks his computer while we talk, and he then tells me whether it is okay or not.

When I first noticed white tea for sale, for example, I inquired of my *internist*, and he immediately responded by telling me from memory what the anti-oxidant ratings of common teas are.

As the years went by, a *blood pressure* medication has been added, one for *cholesterol*, and one to keep my *blood sugar level* in check. Obviously, my *liver* and *kidneys* were aging and needed help. I stopped by an herb store I respect, looking for what to add to my diet to help my *liver* and *kidneys*. The well informed shop clerk suggested *dandelion*. I added those to my winter tea brew. A mulling spice went on sale one winter. I bought up several bottles. I began tossing mulling spices into my daily winter tea. A routine developed with the approval of my medical team. It was one which still included above threshold pain, especially during hot weather and if I exerted at all.

When I first went into dollar stores, I was amazed at

the wide variety of goods available there. I began buying this and that there. It was a good place to pick up plastic bags and cleaning products for general uses rather than specialized uses. I discovered that soymilk was sold more economically there than at grocery stores.

I seeded an area around my patio with *mint* for summer tea and discovered the *mood elevating* effects of *mint* that have been long known. That is a bit of nostalgia. My mother was a *mint* tea drinker.

I tried *Echinacea* tea at one point when it was on sale and did not experience any beneficial effects, so I did not stick with that.

This and that happened in life, as things do.

Then, I happened to find *chamomile* tea on sale during the winter about three years ago. What the heck. It was a dollar. I would try it—at least to see what it tasted like. I had never had it before.

The *sheep sorrel* tea had stopped my getting *bronchitis* and *sore throats*, but a *flu shot* was still required. I had started asking for a pneumonia vaccination before I turned 50 and had always been refused until after I was put on disability. Then during one hospitalization I was actually asked if I wanted a pneumonia vaccination. I said yes and then explained that I had asked when I was younger but had been refused. The hospital staff informed me that since I had *several diagnosed chronic conditions*, I qualified for a pneumonia vaccination despite still being too young for it based on age. Still, nothing stopped the *common cold*.

At least nothing stopped the *common cold* for me until that first winter when I started having one tea bag of *chamomile* tea each day. That winter I did not catch cold. I decided to continue with the *chamomile* tea experiment, and again I did not catch a cold all the next winter. That was enough to convince me, since I had been having colds my entire life except for those two, consecutive winters.

The tea was still available at the rate of 20 tea bags for a dollar, so when I stopped the *sheep sorrel* tea for the warm months, I continued the *chamomile*. I would dump a tea bag into my bottled water when I went out for the day to flavor the water instead of using the *sheep sorrel*. The *sheep sorrel* was simply more difficult to obtain and slightly more costly. All I intended it to do was give some flavor to the bottled water.

When I did not get a cold that second winter, I changed my normal routine permanently. Ah, ha! I reasoned that I would use the *sheep sorrel* tea during the cold weather and the mint tea during the warm weather and *chamomile* tea year round at $.05 a teabag. During the end of that first summer of drinking *chamomile* tea daily, I noticed that my hand/wrist/forearm were not screaming at me in pain. I began reducing my prescription medications. The second summer of this routine, I found that my right hand/wrist/forearm did not scream at me in pain all summer long.

When I returned to my *orthopedist* to order a new kind of brace that an acquaintance uses and showed to me, I asked my *orthopedist* about *chamomile*. He praised it with some animation. He said that, indeed, it has traditionally been attributed *anti-inflammatory* influences. He approved whole heartedly. Thus, I use the chamomile now with the blessings of my *orthopedist* and *internist*.

Now, I am at the end of the third winter of drinking one teabag of *chamomile* tea almost every day. I still put one tea bag into my bottled water when I go out on errands. When I have no need to go out, I intentionally brew up some most days. When I put the *chamomile* tea bag into my bottled water, the tea is cold brewed. Of course, this does not release all of the flavor, nor all of the color, but it is convenient to me to brew it this way. I have lost my fear of

the discomforts of the common cold, since I have not gotten
one since I started drinking *chamomile* tea daily year round.
Above threshold pain days gradually started declining in
number. My activity level gradually was able to go up.
This resulted in some increases in ability to manage self care
and errands. Chores remained a problem but a problem
which very gradually began to lighten.

I have even seen one other person out in public with a
tea bag cold brewing in a commercial plastic bottle of water.
I've been cold brewing tea that way for about a dozen years.

I am now in the 15th year of my hand/wrist/forearm
injury. For the first dozen years, the conditions were stable
and awful. After the first six years, an effective prescription
medicine was found. Before that, *comfrey* had been of some
assistance. Still, considering everything that had been tried
for a dozen years, little healing had occurred. After the first
six years, physicians were able to mask the pain somewhat,
so that it could be kept below threshold much of the time.
Gabapentin blocked the pain message as it arrived in my
brain. Hot weather and any exertion had continued to be
problems that caused miserable pain of long duration.

Call it coincidence or not; when I started drinking

chamomile tea, the *inflammatory condition* seemed to start reversing. However, the salutatory relief might have been from the *cayenne* peppers I had started eating two years earlier. I was given five cayenne pepper trees and still have one of their descendents plants, which provides me with new peppers all summer. I keep the excess in the freezer, so I have these peppers to eat in stews and soups and in noodle dishes year round. I put one or two *cayenne peppers* cut up into any pot of stew, soup, noodle dish, or rice dish that I boil.

Chamomile and *Cayenne* have been studied scientifically. *Chamomile* has several substances that are scientifically known for reducing inflammation. One designated *-a-bisabolo* is among the most powerful antiflammatories known to science. *Capsaicin* found in *cayenne* has been shown scientifically to block pain messages from traveling through the nerves. If the *cayenne* contributed to the cure of my arms, I believe it was in conjunction with *chamomile*. My physical system seems to respond well to *-a-bisabolo* and *capsaicin*.

Some people seem unaware that when effective natural compounds are found to treat illness, commercial firms can chemically synthesize those same compounds, test them, and attempt to sell them on the market. This is one of the roles of contemporary chemistry. Chemists analyze naturally occurring compounds, synthesize these, and then supervise animal trials first and then human clinical trials through which FDA approval is sought for commercial distribution.

I was able to reduce my dependence on *gabapentin, lideocaine,* and *declofenac.* However, I keep them in reserve for when I exert a bit too much and bring on a flare up.

Oh, a small ache is still there, but I can ignore it most of the time. If I misbehave and overdo, I can and do still get *neural spasms* that paralyze the right fingers and thumb for a period of time — generally but not always less than an hour. This spring I learned that I am one of those people who has to regulate my life with my brain and not act or react on impulse, emotion, or intuition. I am one of those people who has to design a life pattern and not just do whatever I feel like at a given moment. For me, this is self protective, not constraining.

I really do enjoy working as hard as I can, and I enjoy feeling strong emotions, but my mind has to take care of my body and keep it out of trouble, out of pain, and out of anxiety.

At a health fair once, a nurse demonstrating a life expectancy, computer program stated that the longer one lives the longer one is predicted to live because those who have survived have developed survival skills that continue to be of assistance.

We learn: a reasonable number of calories, moderate sugar, no added salt, vitamins, water to flush out toxins, sunlight, exercise, at least 6 hours of sleep a night, not making a habit of 12 hour work days, nor 7 day work weeks, etc., etc.

I monitor to determine whether continuing to drink chamomile tea will in the future completely eliminate all of the pathological inflammatory symptoms in my arms. The really unexpected aspect psychologically is that when the pain is entirely gone in my right arm, it is as though a constant companion is absent. How odd is that? My conscious mind has to remind my emotions that it is really fine for that constant condition of pain to be missing! It is almost as though the body interprets the absence of enduring pain as a symptom of danger — as it actually would be in the case of threats like frostbite, for example, as I understand it.

If I overuse my right hand, it still flares up once in a while. The memory of the cruel levels of pain remains very fresh. However, I no longer have to visualize the rest of my life as being crippled by one arm not functioning, nor as being controlled and dominated by cruel levels of pain.

The maintenance prescriptions cannot be the reason. I leave those in the bottles. The *lidocaine patches* are still useful on occasions of overuse.

What amazes me is how much better my arms have gotten since I began adding the *chamomile* tea to my daily diet. I own **no** *chamomile* tea stock, nor stock in any company associated with *chamomile* tea, so I am not disclosing this to see any stock soar.

Personally, I have not been getting colds either, although I have discussed this with one woman who says she drinks *chamomile* tea regularly and continues to catch colds. This result reinforces the long standing impression that traditional herbs do seem to have a tendency to be metabolized somewhat differently by different people. What patent pharmaceuticals strive for is a near uniform and near universal reaction.

It seems to me that it might be worthwhile for those with *inflammatory* conditions to try the herbs that are reported to have traditional reputations as *anti-inflammatories* while not abandoning scientific, licensed medical advice and scientific, licensed medical approaches. That includes checking with your own medical team for their approval before each and every herb you try out. I certainly would not want to be without modern medicine even though I have experienced it to be resisting rather than facilitating.

I had only known about aspirin and had used that. Even when inflammatory conditions had been explained to me and inflammatory diseases had been explained to me, it took me a long time to get rid of the superstitious belief that the body can heal all of its injuries that result from use rather than from accident events. Americans really are put at risk by the superman / superwoman myths. We cannot do everything. We cannot even do everything that we would like to be able to do. And oh how Americans hate to admit that!

It had not even occurred to me that there existed herbs with traditional reputations as *anti-inflammatories*. I ought to have consulted my physicians about them much earlier than I did and methodically tried them one by one earlier than I did. I discovered *chamomile* simply as the result of a dollar store sale long after I had given up hope of ever finding a cure or exercising my way into a cure.

Everyone had had the attitude that the body has a natural inclination to heal itself. One of my hand specialists had, indeed, stated that *the body heals to a level of use.* If an injured part is not used during the healing process, it heals up stiff rather than flexible.

A nurse had told me that when the body is working on healing, it has to work on healing all of its injuries at the same time. She had said that the body does not heal its wounds in sequence, concentrating on one and then another and then another. The body works simultaneously on healing all of its ailments. One injury does not heal first because it is the most important; it heals first because it is the smallest.

I had not seen any indication from my body that it had the ability to heal my arms prior to my using the *chamomile*. Even the *comfrey* had brought on only slight improvements.

5. *Dueling Medical Reports*

Along the way during these most recent fifteen years, I have learned some unexpected things about American society and American culture. Without overhauling the legal system of all 50 states and the federal court system, the United States is incapable of going to a single payer system of health care. The United States medical and legal systems depend on dueling medical reports in all categories of personal injury litigation. If there is a vehicular accident, if there is a slip and fall, if there is an on the job injury, the plaintiff and the defendant depend on independent medical reports as evidence in litigation.

Personal injury lawyers have a reputation for sending their clients to their doctors. That is generally intoned in a derogatory manner. The term 'their doctors' simply refers to the licensed physicians that attorneys have found to provide adequate medical reports for plaintiffs in the past and, perhaps, wait for payment until there is either a settlement or an award as the result of a trial.

Personal injury attorneys know from experience which local physicians are *plaintiff doctors* and which ones are *defense doctors.* Members of the legal profession know who are the *plaintiff lawyers* and who are the *defendant lawyers.* Law firms which customarily work for defendant corporations know who are the *defense doctors.* These are only secret from the public at large.

American law is an *advocate system,* and there are members of the medical profession who line up for or against workers and for or against employers. Insurance always lines up on its own side, which is generally aligned with employers to keep insurance costs down. The terms *keeping insurance costs down* and *preventative medicine* also refer to preventing litigation awards from going to those who are ill or injured or who claim to be ill or injured. There is nothing wrong with keeping insurance costs down and preventative medicine as long as patient needs are served.

Corporations brag about *capturing profits* and *outsourcing costs. Outsourcing* medical costs means shifting injured employees off business and corporate health insurance and onto either Workers Comp., Medicare, or Medicaid. Because businesses have to contribute to

Workers Compensation on a basis that takes into consideration how many of their own employees draw benefits from Workers Comp., businesses prefer to shift the medical costs to Medicaid or Medicare. Even private schools and non-profits pay into Workers Compensation. Both Workers Comp. and group health insurance premiums go up when the employees they cover make claims and receive funds or have their health care providers receive funds.

The goal of tying low premiums to group whose covered members make few or no claims on Workers Comp. and group health insurance started out by providing incentives to businesses to provide healthy working conditions. Over the decades, employers have discovered that they can also keep their benefits costs down by stringently defending against litigation filed by employees who do claim to have been harmed by their working conditions. Such stringent defense is now widely and deeply woven into the texture of American case law. The cry that periodically goes up against the magnitude of awards to plaintiffs in personal injury litigation is a cry that translates into juries and judges or juries having found someone responsible for a dire injury to someone else.

How much should an employer have to pay, if 60 hour workweeks result in a repetitive motion injury to an employee's hand, wrist, and/or forearm such that the employee can no longer feed or clothe himself or herself? The remaining hand cannot always do the job for the entire remaining lifetime of that person. The remaining arm can be seen to sustain *collateral injury* from having to take on the work of two hands. How much in settlement or in a trial judgment does it take to keep such a person from becoming dependent on the taxpayers for their survival?

One reason that Medicare and Medicaid increase year over year is that business has gotten better and better at dumping their own injured employees onto the taxpayer. Severely injured employees tend to have to stop working, and when they do, they no longer have access to their employment based health care insurance. Sometimes there is a spouse who is working who has health care insurance, but this generally does not allow coverage for medical conditions that already exist, when the injured spouse is enrolled after losing his or her own job.

The process of shifting injured employees onto Medicaid and Medicare is done through dueling medical reports and by injured former employees having to consume almost all of their own assets before Medicaid and Medicare social safety nets will grant benefits. Both Medicaid and Social Security Disability have *means tests*. Having a house and an older car are usually permitted. Bank accounts, investments, and pension plans may have to be consumed entirely except for a few thousand dollars in a person's savings before Medicaid or Medicare benefits will start. Neither Medicaid nor Medicare benefits will automatically keep a person from bankruptcy or homelessness. Neither Medicaid nor Medicare provides mortgage or rent payments or real estate taxes. Neither Medicaid nor Medicare prevents health service providers from filing suit against the ill person's financial assets to satisfy co-pays.

Social Security also depends upon dueling medical reports. In addition to the medical reports that an individual provides from his or her own physicians, Social Security sends the individual to a physician that Social Security selects and pays for an *outside opinion*. The physician that Social Security pays for such a report can find the individual disabled and the result be that Social Security still denies the individual's claim for benefits. For Social Security to allow the claim, the disability has to be one for which there exists a Social Security *diagnostic code*. The Social Security paid physician knows those codes. The individual's own physician(s) might not!

For example, all my physicians finally settled down to agreeing that my diagnosis was *de Quervain's tenosynovitis*. At that time, that condition did not have a Social Security disability *diagnostic code*. When that happens, everyone has to wait around for another diagnosis that does have a Social Security *diagnostic code* to develop as the result of the initial injury before Social Security and Medicare come into play. Even if a physician is sympathetic to the patient's circumstances, the physician's hands are tied, if the patient's condition or conditions do not have Social Security *diagnostic codes*. Worse than that—a patient may not know to consult a physician who is knowledgeable about Social Security *diagnostic codes*. One of the values of an attorney who does an active practice in Social Security Disability claims is that such an attorney generally is well informed about which local physicians know the Social Security *diagnostic codes*. The code numbers are published, not classified information.

Also, Social Security currently only pays monthly amounts ranging from under $600/month to about

$2,100/month, depending on work record. Those who would otherwise qualify for the $2,000 range are generally the same people who would have to sell off the most assets before passing the means tests required to receive Social Security Disability. While Social Security Retirement does not currently have a means test, disability certainly does. Thus, receiving Medicare as a disabled person does have a means test already.

Unemployment insurance will not necessarily fill the gap, if Social Security refuses to grant a disability claim. Social Security declaring a person to be able bodied does not control what Unemployment Insurance decides on the same issue. A state unemployment office employee can look and applicant up and down and refuse to accept a claim. How many American employees know what to do, if a state unemployment office employee without a medical degree tells them that they look too disabled to work?

Americans really ought to realize that when financial planners inform them that they must have enough personal savings to live on for a year, the stark truth might be five years.

And the reality can get worse than that.

If an employee reports on a doctor's intake form that the exam is needed for a job injury, the doctor or hospital may elect to delay billing the employee health insurance for the exam or treatment and allow the expenses to accrue without transferring them to the employee's health insurance and getting the bills paid. The bills may add up for years while going unpaid. These can be reported on the patient's credit record as delinquent.

The medical office staff might even say that the reason they are accumulating the unpaid billings is to avoid the medical office having to pay the funds back to the health insurance company when the injury is settled through Workers Compensation or through litigation. So the medical bills build up and build up and build up as personal debt and go on the injured person's credit report as unpaid.

Things can get worse than this!

What the medical staff may not be so forthcoming about is that most employer paid for health insurance will never pay, if a bill is not presented to them for payment within two years. Injury litigation may take much longer than two years to resolve or appeal. Thus, while the disabled employee wends his or her way through the legal system, *all* of person's accruing medical bills for care of the injury are getting shifted off of the employer health care group benefits by the terms of the insurance policy. That policy is a contract between the employer and the insurance company, not the employee. At two years or so (depending on the exact terms of the insurance policy), that door slams shut against the former employee.

At that point, the former employee may be out of work, still disabled, and living on...what?

If there is not litigation, the former employee can become financially crippled by medical debt despite having been covered by an employment based, group health program at the time of injury and at the time of treatment!

This is part of the meaning behind employers *outsourcing expenses* to the taxpayer in order to *capture profits*. Not only the former employee suffers. The taxpayer picks up the tab in a wide variety of ways.

The propaganda is that American homeless are alcoholics and/or drug addicts and released felons. Most of them are divorced. Most of them claim that they ought to be on Social Security Disability. Almost all of them are former employees. Where did they come from? Most of them lost health, job, property, and family. Most of them claim it was from a back injury or a shoulder injury or the like. Go talk to them. Volunteer at your local soup kitchen. Take a casserole over to your local homeless shelter. Sit down at a table and ask, 'How are you doing.' Then just shut up and sit there and be willing to listen. They might not talk to you the first time you ask. Go back and do it again until they do. Then you will learn some core information about how American culture functions.

If you ever wonder why the prison statistics show over a 40% recidivism rate within three years of release, consider that prisons provide medical care, food, and shelter. Not everyone is willing to live homeless on the streets. Other than not having access to women, prison conditions tend to be superior to homelessness. Unless group housing in a halfway house is part of a parole program, those paroled have at least one incentive for violating the terms of their release and returning to prison: it is easier than committing another crime, getting caught, and going through yet another trial — if the primary goal of the criminal is food, shelter, and/or medical care.

Some of those really stupid crimes you hear about in

the media news are stupid crimes *on purpose.* There are American citizens who *want* to be caught in the act and sent to jail or prison and given medical care and food and shelter. If Workers Comp. turns them away, if Unemployment Insurance turns them away, if Social Security Disability turns them away, if Medicaid turns them away…where do you suppose that they *will* go?

Some live in tents hidden away somewhere and collect food stamps and beg on the streets. Others rob a convenience store, bank, business, car, or home. Some get good at it. Some do it in order to get caught and taken in out of the cold. Check the crime statistics during the winter as opposed to those in the summer, if you don't believe this line of argument.

Genuinely mentally ill people were forced out of mental hospitals in the 20th century because it was noticed that genuinely desperate people who were unwilling to commit a crime were able to fake mental illness symptoms in order to avoid homelessness. Statistics were kept that proved that medical expenses went down when large numbers of formerly hospitalized persons were deinstutionalized. The truly mentally ill were unable to coordinate medical care as good as they had received in the mental hospitals, and the desperate who had faked symptoms either became criminals, homeless, or developed some other coping strategy. Non-profits developed to attempt to rescue the truly mentally ill and get them situated outside of hospitals — with mixed success and failure.

Contemporary statistics prove that it costs about $200,000 to house the mentally ill in a private hospital for a year, $150,000 in a state hospital, close to $40,000 in a group home, and less than $10,000 in public housing. Prison care for convicts runs close to $40,000 in states outside of the Southeast, and drug halfway houses can run into that range, depending on the professional staffing by health care providers, including social workers. Some of the over 50 billion annual cost to states for prison expenses could be reduced by providing group homes and medical care for mentally or physically disabled ex-cons outside the prison system where they would be less expensive and more likely to avoid recidivism.

Veterans who become disabled after service still apply to the V.A. for assistance with survival care.

Recently, there was legislation proposed to limit mental illness diagnostic codes to those who test as imbeciles — baring the wider array of mental health diagnostic codes.

Getting an on the job injury that does not result from a specific, witnessed event can really be life threatening in a nation that throws its disabled workers onto the garbage heap. Certainly, employers don't want to hire anyone who has sustained a previous injury, since that person might sustain reinjury. In capitalist America, it is not wonder that employees litigate.

Dueling medical reports can be a life or death matter.

6. *Softening-Up Litigants*
for Settlement

Despite 70% of the lawyers in the world being in practice in the United States, an injured employee might not be able to find an attorney. At least since California attorneys L. Jacoby and S. Meyers broke the advertising ban in law practice, the public can go to the yellow pages and to online search engines to find an attorney — and one who offers a free initial consultation. Those are usually but not exclusively by telephone. Keep calling until an attorney who is comfortable in employment law takes the case. That is the first stage you have to go through. The difficulty *softens you up* for settlement. In the meantime, open a file to keep all of your medical records. That file perhaps should be a box rather than a folder.

Union members turn to their unions. Professor ought to have memberships in AAUP, since AAUP benefits generally include providing an attorney in the instance of faculty/administration conflict. If you have AAUP membership, you're probably not going to be overworked into disability in the first place because college administrations are frequently aware of AAUP practices.

In some professions, injured members reduce their own scheduled hours and/or hire in a junior staff member to mentor in order to get the physical work done while the professional in charge continues to provide supervision and judgment required under law.

We might ask why the United States has 70% of the lawyers in the world, anyway. What do Americans fight so much about. We all know the answer to that question: money. In estates, in divorces, in personal injury, in environmental lawsuits, in criminal cases, in most conflicts involving lawyers, money is at issue on one side even if it is not on the other side.

Understand that your employer is/will be fighting you over money, if your disability claim is contested. There certainly are employers who cooperate with Workers Compensation claims, especially if their rate of injury is very low and they have been paying into the system for many years. Good employers with low injury rates are known to foster injured employees and help them through the process. The worse the employer's record, the more they are paying into Workers Compensation, and the more they will fight claims.

If your hand/wrist/arm is injured in such a manner that it is difficult for you to carry, difficult for you to drive, and difficult for you to perform self-care, ask your medical team to prescribe a wheelchair for you. If your physician tells you to stop carrying your briefcase or purse, ask for a wheelchair to carry it for you. Wheelchairs are not generally granted for hand/wrist/arm injuries. However, how else are you going to carry things and avoid collateral injury to your other arm? Ask yourself, 'If my leg or legs were injured, would I have difficulty performing this task?' Driving and carrying are certainly activities that are impacted by hand/wrist/arm injuries as are leg injuries.

When your supervisor or a person from human resources asks you the required questions about what assistive devices you require under the Americans with Disabilities Act, ask for a wheelchair, if carrying is a typical part of your job, and you have a hand/wrist/arm injury. They might not like it, and you might not like the idea of it. However, it might save your career. You might only have

12 weeks off in which to heal. After that, you might be fired.

If you consider that Workers Compensation, Social Security Disability, and Unemployment Insurance might all deny your claims, what are you going to do in pain and out of work, if you don't solve the problem of your injury quickly?

Having to sit in a wheelchair with soften you up and soften up your employer for settlement. It is a strategy that pushes both sides, not just one.

There is considerable disillusionment that occurs on both sides during litigation in the United States. Many members of the public believe that settlement of an injury lawsuit depends on the merits of the case, and they may believe that if their physician or physicians say they are permanently injured that a high recovery should be rather automatic. However, the overall medical record of treatment can be a determining factor. Some attorneys will candidly report that a settlement offer is frequently calculated at a multiple of the medical bills outstanding.

Consider the view of the liability insurance company that is looking at a medical record of $10,000 for one year's treatment of an injury. Consider the view of the liability insurance company that is looking at a medical record of $200,000 for one year's treatment of an injury. If you were the executive in charge of calculating the settlement offer to be made, what would you offer to the first plaintiff and what would you offer to the second plaintiff for lifetime care?

Injured persons who believe that settlement is on the merits as opposed to settlement being on the record of medical costs don't necessarily understand the system of American law. An employer's basic goal may be to have you offered just enough for you to be able to leave the community and have everyone you worked with forget about you. That sum differs markedly from what it might take you to live on for 20 years.

Also, find out if your pension plan has a disability pay-out and the terms for qualifying for that.

Some people with personal injuries may come around to being willing to settle on almost any terms. They may settle without taking into consideration that the medical bills that have been accruing are still hanging out there. To get a bill covered by a settlement, the person's attorney has to have a copy of the bill. Some might have gotten lost and remain unpaid. Financial ruin can still follow a personal injury settlement. Unless the settlement negotiations are conducted properly, an injured former employee can settle litigation and still be bankrupted by outstanding medical bills. A competent plaintiff lawyer will accumulate all of the medical record, including all of the medical bills that are turned in to him or her.

Settlements are usually conducted based on the size of the accumulated medical bills and the plaintiff's attorney's fees, not on gestimates of how long the plaintiff might take to recover, if at all.

Patients who have attempted to minimize their medical expenses rather than maximize their medical care are, therefore, disadvantaged in litigation.

The defendant vehicle driver or sidewalk owner or employer will have the injured person ordered to report to defendant selected physicians for opposing medical reports. Naïve patients might believe that one or the other of the doctors must be accepted as correct *when, procedurally, it may be the cost of the entire accumulated medical record which is the decisive factor in determining the settlement offer to be made or accepted.*

Thus, it is basically unreasonable to worry about the

findings by the opposition physician or physicians. They are consulted to disprove the plaintiff's statements, not to prove them. Opposition medical staff is a part of the advocacy system. Each side is entitled to advocates.

If there were to be a single provider health care system in the United States, how would parties to personal injury litigation obtain the required dueling medical reports currently used by the plaintiffs and the defendants? Employees who are terminated could continue to get uninterrupted medical care, producing a comprehensive medical record despite loss of employer paid for health care. Who would employers go to for defendant medical reports, if a governmental, single provider health care system went into place? Employers are desperate to maintain the existence of physicians that they can pay for the medical reports that employers need to duel with employees who claim injury on the job.

A single payer health care system in the United States would as a system tend to soften-up employers to settle with their injured employees. Better than that, it would motivate employers to provide healthier working conditions, especially with regard to working hours and the severity of labor tasks.

Employers can now *outsource* injured employee care to Medicare or Medicaid even while Workers Compensation claims are pending. Employers can even *outsource* injured employee care to the jail and prison systems, if a former employee crumbles that far.

A government paid for single provider health care system might have a natural inclination to provide medical reports that hold employers responsible for their employees rather than continuing to tolerate the business *outsourcing costs* to the government for former employee maintenance. Social Security Disability payouts would be reduced in that instance, so would Medicaid costs, and penal system costs. At current payouts, Social Security payouts are about $7,200 to $24,000 a year, depending on the person's former contributions into the system. At current government costs, a year in group home or prison costs around $40,000, depending on the state in which the group home or prison is operated.

As mentioned previously, according to current practice, state unemployment offices can decide that an employee is *disabled* and unable to collect unemployment benefits simultaneously with federal Social Security

Disability deciding that an employee is *not* disabled and unable to collect disability benefits. Simultaneously, both safety nets are allowed to reach contradictory decisions, excluding unemployed persons from the protection of those safety nets. This is nonsensical. Either unemployment benefits ought to apply or disability benefits ought to apply through both systems.

This contradiction is one of the practices at the core of States' Rights vs. Federal Rights. Government gains by barring unemployed citizens from collecting on either their unemployment benefits or their disability benefits. Where does this leave the everyday citizen worker? They must consume almost all of their own resources, including their retirement nest egg and then qualify for Medicaid. There is not a disability test for Medicaid, only an impoverishment test and demonstrated need for medical care.

The process of *softening-up* the injured, making them more agreeable to settlement on almost any terms offered, can include abandonment by family, including divorce.

Considerable funding is expended to spread propaganda that homelessness is a product of drug and alcohol abuse and to obscure the extent to which drug and alcohol abuse are self medicating for pain resulting from job injuries — backaches, knee pain, shoulder pain, loss of family ties, and the like. Men are particularly vulnerable to self medicating with drug and alcohol abuse; American culture does not do a good job of training its male population in self care.

Some families hold together, and the able bodied spouse takes on increased burdens. Some families go to pieces when medical bills threaten the family home, for example. An injured man might even agree to give up his home to his wife and children through a divorce property settlement agreement rather than see his children go out onto the streets with him after he in injured on the job and has run up high medical bills.

Irritability can be the first symptom of pain that presents itself — even before pain above threshold is recognized. Men do not always recognize that they might need medical care when they become irritable, but if they do not, they can end up losing their jobs and their families. When a knowledgeable physician asks them what is bothering them, a man might report that his back is bothering him or his arm, leading to prescriptions that might be of considerable assistance.

Family problems that tend to get blamed on women working are sometimes family problems that result in a mother having to go to work to support her children to keep the family home while the former husband and father in physical pain becomes a homeless man *in the system*. The phrase *in the system* can refer to Veterans Administration care, homeless shelter care, penal care, drug rehab care, and a variety of other rather shredded social safety nets.

During injury litigation, stressing families until they fragment is a significant benefit to employers, since an injured employee or former employee who lacks the support of a family is an injured employee or former employee who is less likely to be able to withstand the ordeal of waiting out the years before reaching trial. Thus, an injured employee or former employee who has a supportive family is a plaintiff who is less likely to settle litigation for a low sum.

The Workers Compensation system is the one that is supposed to be working to prevent employee catastrophe from on-the-job injuries. Workers Comp. tends to work best with specific accident incidents — with witnesses. It works less well without witnesses to a discrete event.

Workers Compensation works least well with repetitive motion injuries. Even there, it functions better with factory workers than professional and managerial staff. These categories are mistakenly thought to have job functions that are not physically demanding but are rather intellectually demanding. Across the board, Americans underestimate how constantly their hands are required during post-industrial employment.

Medical specialists can be very tightly tied into the state Workers Compensation system. If they are really good physicians, then they can get people repaired and healed up and back to work, and Workers Compensation is very interested in that. However, not all former employees can be repaired and healed.

Some of employees injured on the job have to go out of state in order to get honest medical reports as a result of excellent in-state physicians being economically dependent on Workers Compensation for their own livelihood. After all, the more medical reports a physician writes that favor the injured employee or former employee, the more likely the physician will gain a reputation as being a *plaintiff physician* in the system of dueling medical reports for litigation. The more that happens, the more requests the physician might receive to defer bill collection pending litigation settlement or trial. The more that happens, the less hard cash the physician has coming in to meet his or her own professional and personal expenses day to day.

One *occupational medicine* specialist physician of my acquaintance abandoned the field upon learning that occupational medicine as a specialty holds an anti-employee bias. The occupational specialist physician I personally am acquainted with finally went to work for FEMA, where assisting citizens is better tolerated.

Without physicians that employers pay and physicians that employees can hire independent of employers' money, United States personal litigation cannot obtain the medical reports current legal procedures require. Plaintiffs get medical reports that state that they are injured and why. Defendants get medical reports that state that while the plaintiff may experience subjective pain and may or may not be injured, the alleged injury cannot be the fault of the defendant, especially the defendant employer. Emphasis is put on how *subjective* pain is. There is no specific laboratory test for a specific chemical that will conclusive inform all sides what the patient's pain level is.

The defendant has to withstand the duration and the

expense of the litigation — which many cannot withstand. Those who cannot stand up under the current system do *not* get justice in the courts; they may never see the inside of the courtroom. Some have family, a union, or a professional association who will foot the legal expenses. Even college and university professors have access to this — if only they knew the American Association of University Professors has had a tradition of providing free legal assistance to their members who get into legal tangles with their administrations.

Employers rely on the harsh consequences that result from employee ignorance. All of the harsh consequences *soften-up* the plaintiff for settlement. Employers don't have to know the breaking points of any individual employee's circumstances. Employers are able to strain them all. Many employers will simply say, 'No,' as long as possible to as many requests as the injured employee or former employee makes.

Sometimes plaintiff lawyers inform their clients that the role of the client is to say, 'No,' to settlement until his/her attorney advises otherwise.

But there are employees and former employees who are so seriously injured that they cannot sustain themselves during the contemporary process of litigation. Some of these are so injured as to have to consume all of their assets. They, indeed, can end up on Medicaid and may very well go from Medicaid to Medicare and remain a burden to the taxpayer for life *rather than becoming a burden to stockholders, rather than becoming a drag on the bottom line.* American personal injury litigation is imperfect. It is a spotty, hit or miss system. Some of the homeless are people who have gotten crushed in the hit or miss system.

People enter the professions in attempts to avoid such a fate. People enter unions in attempts to avoid such fates. However, it isn't really *fate.* It is social engineering that is designed to consume employees as objects and favor the top of the hierarchy being able to buy yachts and send their offspring to elite colleges and elite universities and to pay for $100,000 weddings, country club memberships, mansions, etc., etc. Some of these luxuries go to foreign corporate heads at the expense of American employees and American taxpayers.

The United States is not only a nation of poor immigrants who pulled themselves up by their bootstraps and hard work. The United States is also a culture built up by formerly aristocratic immigrants who in their hearts and souls continue to believe that serfdom and peasantry are valid and desirable conditions to subject upon others. Dehumanizing terms continue to be applied to the laboring pubic — such terms as *worker bees*. There are some managers who feel they ought to have no more concern for an employee's arm or leg than for the wing of a honey bee.

An increasingly large number of Generation X women are going into business management where they may find that neither being a professional, nor being in a union will be of any assistance to them. When Generation X agitates for the elimination of Social Security and Medicare benefits, they argue for the elimination of safety nets members of their own generation are fast approaching needing. Greenspan and others are on the record, stating that when Medicare reaches crisis, there are plans to merge it with Medicaid and apply a means test to retirement access to Medicare in addition to the already existing means test for access to Medicare through Social Security Disability benefits. These intentions are already being voiced by some in the daily media. It is an old idea.

More of the middle class than at present will be

required to consume all of their assets prior to obtaining any access to safety nets, especially medical benefit safety nets that already shred to pieces upon impact. Already we have telling statistics. In the 'Great Generation,' 17% did not retire. In the 'Baby Boom' generation, 25% are not planning on retiring — ever. For 'Gen X' is it going to be 35%? Is retirement gradually going to go out of existence?

If one of the definitions of slavery is having to work 12 hours a day, if another definition of slavery is having to work 7 days a week, is not being able to retire — ever — another definition of slavery?

On the most basic level, there is huge cultural conflict between two vast demographics in the American population. One vast segment of the population really does believe and feel and expect that the proper role for all professionals is to serve the functions of a nurturing parent and an excellent school teacher: 1) have a strong interest in the well being of the member of the public and 2) problem solve for the member of the public and 3) foster the growth/improvement of the member of the public. Another vast segment of the population really does believe and feel and expect Social Darwinism to play out: survival of the fittest within a framework of conflict. Social Darwinists accept the use of neglect and exploitation in social and civic interaction. Anyone who does not protect himself or herself from Social Darwinism is probably in for a great deal of trouble from its adherents.

Each profession has its own code of ethics. An individual profession's code of ethics might approve of behaviors that the general public might find very, very surprising. I have certainly been surprised by the code of ethics of my profession. At a public presentation before a university faculty group, I heard a leader in the profession asked about to whom professors owed ultimate responsibility. When university administrators and the student body were in conflict, are professors supposed to do what is best for the administration or what is best for the student body? Of course, the option of doing what was best for the faculty was not even raised! Neither was doing what was best for the individual faculty member!

The leader in the profession of being university professor had an immediate and precise answer. He stated categorically that university professors have a professional responsibility to do what is best for the entire community. The reply was *not* what was best for the academic community but what was best for the *entire* community. That includes the neighborhood, city, and county where the university is located. It can also include geographical regions that are made up of more than one county. Included in what is best for the entire community is what is best for the faculty and the individual professor. Professors, by career choice, are not required to be martyrs. Being a martyr is a different career choice.

What happens to members of the public who expect to be nurtured and fostered by all members of all of the professions? They aren't! Well, they aren't unless they have ample funds with which to pay for every service they believe they require or every service they want.

Attorneys and physicians are not responsible for solving all of the public's problems. Attorneys and physicians are responsible for earning their fees by attempting to solve their client's problems. An injured employee who goes to a physician who is retained to write the report the employer is paying for is going to a physician *whose professional responsibility is to solve the employer's problem. The injured employee is not going to that physician for treatment.* This distinction can be very difficult for members of the public to comprehend. Their lack of comprehension sets them up for settlement — *softens them up.* As disillusionments increase, some plaintiffs desire to settle in order to get out of the litigation system — at almost any cost.

The cultural movement in America towards a single payer health care system is an effort to transform American medicine along the lines of the American public education system and the American civil service system. Pay scales did *not* go down as a result of those two employment transformations. Pay scales when up, so did working conditions. The movement in America towards a single payer health care system does not have the goal of creating socialism or socialist medicine. We don't call the public education system socialist or socialist education. We don't call public libraries socialist — even though most could not afford to belong if memberships were by private subscription.

Consider your local public library. Do you consider it a socialist enterprise? Yet, if it were a capitalistic, membership club, what do you think your private membership would cost to belong to a private club like that? Would you be willing to pay the kind of dues to borrow books that a private health club charges or what a country club charges for use of those resources? We don't have to label as 'socialism' every cultural change that we decide to make together.

As it is, medical care is certainly rationed for at least the poorer 20% of the nation's population. In addition to that, employee group health plans do ration care in ways that the employees do not understand. For example, most employees don't realize that if they are injured at work, their physicians might refuse to submit bills to the group health plan. If the employees submit the bills to their human resources department and get checks drawn, the patients still cannot force the medical providers to cash the checks during pending litigation.

What we have within our *dueling medical reports* system of law and medicine, our two or more year system of *softening-up* plaintiffs before even getting to a settlement conference or before a jury is a system that bankrupts many patients, some hospitals, and few physicians. Hospitals get bankrupted because most states require that they see anyone who comes in the door, regardless of insurance or lack of insurance. In France, hiring wet nurses for infants used to bankrupt some mothers and fathers. At that time, the wet nurse system was thought to be necessary in France. Although the United States claims to have the best medicine in the world, there is a possibility that if it does, it does so *despite* the way the current medical system is organized and *not because* of the way the current medical system is organized.

Actually, in the United States, health care is currently rationed by demonizing the disabled and the impoverished, including children. The disabled and impoverished are largely excluded from what the middle class considers a standard level of health care. The first way the disabled are excluded is by the paperwork required to qualify for any benefits at all. Truly disabled cannot function well enough to process the paperwork and if a family member or human resources staff member does not process the claims, sometimes the disabled have to attempt to survive until they are hospitalized and hospital social workers get benefit paperwork initiated.

The long term disabled and the impoverished depend upon the charity of individual physicians and upon largely volunteer health clinics. Specialists who list with Medicaid can have their practices overwhelmed, resulting in their withdrawing from listing. Also, Medicaid might demand that anyone in that system travel 100 miles to see a specialist of any kind. The only way to be certain of being seen quickly under Medicaid is to go to the emergency room. Hospitals that have to deal with that can fail and close and leave an entire community without hospital care as a result of how much lower Medicaid payments are than Medicare or private insurance.

The current system of medical care in the United States quickly impoverishes members of the middle class who develop a really serious medical condition, and those people fall out of the middle class. In fact, the majority of Americans can only count on receiving excellent medical care during their prime working years — when they least need it. The wealthy, professionals, managers, and union members receive good health care as do their spouses and their children, but the majority of Americans do not.

Communications professionals know as a result of their research that people believe more and more what is repeated to them more and more. To get Americans to believe they have a really excellent health care system all that is required is telling them over and over that they have an excellent health care system! University researchers have found this to be true in study after study for fifty years. Research participants will ignore the evidence of their own direct experience, and they will report what they have been told, instead.

Some employees do so until they are without family, without home, and without funds. By the time they discover reality, they are very much *softened-up* for settlement—and perhaps at values that result in their becoming a burden on the taxpayer rather than dragging down the employer's bottom line.

I have learned to apply the following reality test to any political argument I hear or read:

> Is this argument attempting to persuade me and others that those who **have** must be protected?

> Is this argument attempting to persuade me and others that those who **don't have** must be protected?

Logically, those who **have** really don't require additional protection from starvation and exposure and neglect. They can buy food, housing, and care. Logically, those who **don't have** are the ones who are vulnerable to dying from starvation, exposure, or neglect. The basic argument of the haves is to tell us to let the have nots die, that the have nots are not worthy of our attention, nor worthy of resources. That attitude makes a civilization more and more cruel.

During litigation, the defendant side is unconcerned with how weak the hand is that signs the settlement documents. The defendant side will send fifteen people to a settlement conference to intimidate the plaintiff. It is a statement of, 'All of us are against you and your legal team. How can you expect to win?' In the alternative, the defendant side will send one young attorney whose primary strength is the stamina of youth — the ability to stay at the negotiations table longer than the plaintiff's side.

After all of the *softening-up* process, the plaintiff has to remain tough enough to sit at the table and say, 'No.'

The plaintiff's attorney will eventually say, 'Well, I think we have an agreement finally,' or the judge will indicate that he/she will set the dispute for trial.

Sometimes, plaintiffs don't understand that they simply have to continue to sit at the conference table regardless of the other chaos that is going on.

7. Trends Going Forward

There are measures that employee citizens can take in the attempt to protect themselves, their families, and their lifestyles. One is to avoid buying into the American myth that Americans are Supermen and Superwomen who can do everything that everyone asks of them. Forty hour workweeks are one thing. Thirty-five workweeks are more self-protective. Fifty hour workweeks are unwise. Sixty hour workweeks are foolhardy and abusive or self abusive. Even if a person loves his or her job, rest and recreation are vital. *Rest and recreation are vital even if they seem boring in comparison with the stimulation and the rewards of the job.*

As a society, we also need to stop electing politicians on the basis of their short term memory skills rather than their long term memory skills. An individual with strong short term memory and strong processing memory can perform very well in response to interview questions and can perform very well during debates. They can come up with great sound bites on the spot. At the same time, these same politicians can entirely lack long term memory problem solving ability that is essential in dealing with monitoring and adjusting developing social, cultural, economic, and global patterns. Sound bites can garner votes for politicians who have no ability to solve problems that last longer than a few minutes. Being great under pressure requires more than giving a great performance while the spotlights are on.

As a response to media reports that Generation X wants to destroy Social Security and Medicare, we may well be experiencing Baby Boomers adjusting to that threat by becoming more self-protective in their spending and saving habits. Professional demographers are watching the Baby Boom generation very carefully, and already there are reports that American savings are going up. If Baby Boomers sock away enough cash savings to protect themselves in case the promises of Social Security suddenly vanish after all they have paid in, Baby Boomers will not be doing as much consumer spending while they are socking away private nest eggs. That will mean that the superheated American economy might not return.

If Baby Boomers across the nation stash away savings instead of buying consumer goods with their former confidence, then that will leave Generation X to attempt on their own to supercharge the American economy. Maybe they will prove up to the task, or maybe they will experience physical breakdowns of various sorts as have the generations that have run the American economy before Generation X. History has yet to inform us about the outcomes of these present trends.

What we do know about historical trends in the United States is that since the original days of the colonies and the days of revolution and civil war, there have been the contending populations of those who see people as objects/commodities and those who see people as valuable in and of themselves as human beings. There are those who would discard an injured employee as readily and as totally as tossing out a broken copy machine or computer.

Already it is clearly known that American corporations prefer to hire and retain B students rather than A students. Students who earned their B grades tend to sit at their desks and do their work the way they are told to do it. They have a good accuracy rate and tend to rely on their personal lives for satisfaction. They do not necessarily notice that companies tend to move them every three years, since corporate profits tend to reflect community networking, and community networking produces increased sales for about three years. B students don't tend to notice that corporations are not run for their benefit like the public schools they attended. B students sometimes discover too late or not at all that professional associations exist in a vast variety of fields and offer them some benefits that parallel some union benefits. B students assume the risk of being followers, sometimes with mistaken assumptions.

On the other hand, A students tend to analyze everything and want to improve everything. Corporations do not necessarily want improvement, since that involves change. Change also involves expense and sometimes risk. A students also tend to want to put deep roots into a community and into a profession, making them harder for corporations to dislodge. A students tend to fare better when they are self employed and free to improve society through innovation. A students assume the risks of being leaders.

Young people come out of the high schools and the colleges having almost their entire lifetime of experience within environments that are highly planned, highly structured, and designed for fostering the maximum growth possible within the educational systems budgetary constraints. For months, for years, for decades, most young people go on assuming that the companies for which they work also are designed for the maximum growth of employee potential. As companies resist their A students, the A students tend to learn the truth about corporate organization and either agitate harder for change or bail out, returning to graduate school, retool for an independent profession, or go into consulting.

Eventually, many B students discover that they have to change from one employer to another, from one career track to another, if they wish to keep growing into their potential. Some get lured into dead-ends by the pay scale or the benefit package, assuming it will be theirs until they retire or die. Somewhere about 50, when the costs of their employer paid health premiums shoot up, many B students suddenly begin to wise up and wake up from many of their illusions. For some, that is already too late.

This maturation process and its learning curve account somewhat for why older citizens tend to have a higher voting record than do younger people. As Americans leave school and fend for themselves, they begin to get enough experience for *reality* to shift somewhat for them. B students realize that their bosses don't care about them nearly as much as parents and teachers did. A students stop being the darlings of those who try to lead leaders as they butt heads. At about the time that their college aged children are expecting parents to pay for young adult illusions, the parents begin discovering some paradigm shift illusions of their own.

As in *Death of a Salesman*, not all of those traffic accidents on the highways are, after all, accidents. Road rage is much more that commuter stress! Road rage is also an expression of failed dreams, failed illusions. Taxpayers who are funding *the system* as well as they can figure out how to do it, literally slam into their competition on the roadways—the anonymous *they* who are at fault—other commuter taxpayers just like themselves. Some of those commute *accidents* are self destruction. Insurance companies write checks that provide for the surviving families.

America set up the American system of protecting minor children from the worst rigors of the workplace — with the consequence that American children by and large do not grow up within the commercial workplace. They expect American companies to be run on teamwork principles like schools, but American companies tend to run on other principles. Students who have fortunately selected careers in which there are worker shortages tend to fare better than students who ignore demographic trends and end up in career fields where there is surplus labor — and with that lower wages. No one ever seems to put a copy of *Occupational Outlook* directly into their hands.

Because each individual breaks down differently within a group of overworked coworkers, the toll that overwork takes primarily surfaces within the context of aging or the context of litigation. Each individual's weakest physical system will break down first. One might have a heart attack while another develops carpel tunnel while another develops emotional problems. One employee develops endocrine problems, another gallstones. Each body begins to malfunction according to which of its systems is not able to keep up with the pace, the tension, the hours, or the tasks. As the employee's medical expenses go up for the employer, the employer may decline to invest other funds into that employee — and even reorganize and downsize as a way of cutting out mature *deadwood* in favor of hiring in fresh new graduates. Many employees are tossed out at about 50, when employer paid health insurance premiums tend to go up.

As long as they can collect unemployment, these middle aged employees then get a few additional weeks, months, or years of R & R while they seek to find another niche for themselves within productive employment. They get to practice at leisure with reduced income in preparation for later adjustment to retirement.

People forget that definitions of slavery. People forget to take days off from *chores* in addition to taking days off from *work*. People forget that days *off* are not necessarily for running errands. People forget to rest. For some reason, *many Americans believe that resting means sleeping* and that all waking hours have to be filled with some sort of activity — or some sort of 'productive' activity.

Americans children ask their parents and their teachers, 'When do I know when I'm thirsty? When do I know when I should go to the bathroom?' The answer they tend to get is, 'Your body will tell you.' I remember asking those questions. The answers I got were *wrong*. People can feel thirst from having a high blood sugar level; thirst does not automatically mean dehydration. Also, bladder and bowel movement can be postponed too long and unknowingly. The correct answers are that we should drink approximately eight glasses of water a day and go to the bathroom approximately twenty minutes later and have a bowel movement once a day. *Feeling* thirsty or *feeling* the urge to eliminate is not the essential factor; performing the action is the essential factor.

Professional drivers tend to develop liver and kidney problems either as a result of not taking enough bathroom breaks or from constant vibrations. Medical science cannot isolate those two possibilities within that population, but their findings do indicate that even adults do not necessarily know when they *have* to go to the bathroom.

The right answer also is not that one has to go to the bathroom once in the mid-morning at coffee break time, once at lunch break, and once in the mid-afternoon at coffee break time — although that is a good start.

We are not taught self care very well, and American men are especially not taught self care very well. One of the best ways to learn self care is to take care of someone else or to take care of other people. This is also a way of learning that people are human beings and not things/objects.

Saying or believing 'I'm having a lot of fun working this hard' is not a safe response in the long run.

When my body broke down and medical science was

not able to patch me up, heal me up, and send me back again, I reflected that I had gone into a line of work that markedly differed from that of my ancestors. We had not as a rule been bureaucrats. We called on our medium sized and large muscles more extensively than we called on our small muscles. My selected profession required extensive use of small muscles. My body was not physically adapted for that adequately. I hadn't started out with the right kinds of small muscles for the profession I had selected. I had needed genetically tough, small muscles.

I started asking myself to identify and restrict my use of my hands to medium sized muscle tasks and large muscle tasks — the general kinds of tasks my ancestors had relied on for their survival. When others could not figure out accommodations for my disabilities, nor adaptive technology for my disabilities, I started trying to figure out medium sized muscle and large size muscle ways to accomplish small muscle tasks. The process of attempting to do so was interesting. I also spent considerable time analyzing cultural and economic trends in order to get reoriented to society as a disabled person. That adaptive process has worked to some extent.

The general public seems to believe that when one

becomes disabled, one also becomes stupid. That is not at all true. The general public seems to believe that when one becomes disabled, one also becomes useless and worthless. That also is not true. Some disabled persons get into that condition by being too self sacrificing. That is an attitude to life that is not always rewarded. A self sacrificing attitude is not necessarily respected either, if it is carried forth to a level of disability.

Politicians tend not to mention that the way *entitlements* function in the American economy is to commodify poverty — to turn services to the poor into business. When anti-poverty programs are attacked politically, those attacks are aimed at the *rival businesses* that service. When services are provided to the poor, employees are needed — employees who cannot be recruited by businesses that seek to exploit the poor.

When government funding for poverty programs is attacked, part of the concern is for financing and part of the silent concern is for staffing. Staffing poverty programs generally redirects the efforts of professionals with college educations. There is a lot of competition for this educated 25% of the population. The more job choice this 25% has, the more commercial businesses have to pay to hire them away from public sector and non-profit organization work.

Food Stamps, for example, prevent a large portion of shoplifting and bring paying business into grocery stores. A political attack on Food Stamps also aims at the grocery industry, which would lose business and experienced some elevation in shoplifting. The poor who have access to Food Stamps and charity food banks do not have an incentive to shoplift groceries, nor dig discarded groceries out of dumpsters in order to try to survive adverse circumstances. Having food on the table, they can stay in school longer, if they are children, or job hunt more effectively, if they are unemployed adults. The formerly middle class father gets a breathing space to consider whether there is some business he can start on his own rather than returning to dependency upon an employer. Anti-poverty programs are very political in their far reaching impact.

Anti-poverty housing subsidies underwrite construction of rental housing. Political attacks on housing subsidies are aimed at the real estate industry in addition to being aimed at the poor. Low income housing that becomes available in one community can reduce the crime rate and the criminal population in another community; an alcoholic who is offered low income housing with a subsidy might stay sober indoors away from the public, for example, instead of robbing a liquor store in attempts to cope with homelessness.

Medicaid pays physicians about enough to cover the cost of a clerical worker to process the paperwork, while the physician generally is donating his/her time as charity. Yes, Medicaid pay rates *are* that low. There is such a shortage of physicians willing to do such charity work that Medicaid patients in some areas who need access to some specialties do have to attempt to travel great distances — even into other counties despite the lack of public transportation options — or go without medical care. For the poor, medical care is already tightly rationed — within a system that is dependent upon physician charity.

While there are many additional specialists who are willing to accept one or half a dozen or a dozen charity patients a month, what happens if they list as accepting Medicare is that they are referred *all* of the untreated in their specialty who would otherwise go untreated. This can overwhelm a physician or his/her practice to the financial detriment of that practice and even threaten the financial viability of that medical practice.

One beneficial reform of Medicaid would be to allow physicians to designate how many Medicaid patients they would be willing to accept, so that no one physician would be forced to treat overwhelming numbers of Medicaid patients or not participate at all. However, that is a reform that would be very hard to implement within current operations.

Political attacks on anti-poverty programs are also aimed at non-profits which receive grants to do the work of society that other segments of the economy are not willing to address. With no commodification of poverty, poverty services tend not to fit in well into a capitalist economy.

Non-profits sometimes are vehicles for dedicated individuals to raise money one way in order to support themselves while they are taking care of some need in the world that is not commodified in such a way for the individuals to earn a living by means of the activity. For example, people are willing to pay $100 to attend a party that may cost $25 per person to arrange. Then $75 can go to paying the salary of someone to run a community service non-profit. Another example is that it might cost $25 to register for a walk or run to benefit the homeless, including receiving an event tee shirt that costs $8 to produce, while the remaining $17 goes to services for the homeless. The selling of one product by the non-profit can raise money to pay for the part of the project that the public refuses to fund directly.

Political attacks on anti-poverty funding sometimes assert the differing needs of differing states and are extensions of the centuries old conflict between States Rights and federal policies. States and state politicians who assert that their populations have needs that do not match federal policies are just that: states that have population policies that do not match federal population policies. The differences can be in attitudes toward race or gender or age or ethnicity. Federal policies are reached by national, representative consensus. One can understand the federal government not wanting to fund standards which disagree with the national consensus. Some states want their populations to have more than federal standards fund. In that instance, states can do so with their own funds.

Some states want segments of their populations to have less than federal standards mandate for federal funds being used. One is entitled to ask why states would want any segment of their population to receive less than federal policies will fund. As I understand it, some federal programs require states to contribute a portion in order to receive federal funds. Some states may really want the federal funds without putting in the state contribution. However, the question is whether it is fair to taxpayers in other states to carry the entire federal financial load for states which are unwilling to have their state taxpayers contribute to the maintenance of their necessitous fellow state residents.

The single health care provider system threatens to change the commodification of poverty produced through the injuries of employees. Not only could a single payer health care system shift the responsibilities for injured employees back onto the profits of the employers, a single payer health care system could increase the percentage of intact families and reduce the number of people willing to commit stupid crimes for the purposes of getting fundamental needs met by becoming jailed or imprisoned.

A single health care provider system would force systemic change throughout American capitalism and the way capitalism structures personal and family life. A single health care provider system would also cause restructuring economic practices in the United States. Those who benefit most from the current system are the ones digging in their heals and their claws to resist a shifting of resources towards the remainder of the members of the shared economy.

The reason they want change to be channeled through existing private medical practice and existing insurance companies is that they vehemently want the medical reports that they can buy though that advocacy system against their on the job injured employees. The federal government knows already that it cannot nationalize private medical practices, but government has to have a way to keep hospitals from failing despite the poor using emergency rooms as their last resort for medical care.

Certainly, the government as health care provider could better defend its own interests by shifting the burden of injured employee needs back onto exploitive employers, thus keeping those costs out of the Medicaid, Medicare, and Social Security Disability systems. Employers would then have to price goods and services in such a way as to allow for non-injurious working conditions on the job. Prices of goods and services would change. Consumer costs would adjust for those consumers who have an interest in those goods and services. Businesses would no longer tend to *capture profits* and *outsource costs* when those costs came to employee health and maintenance needs. Businesses would be forced to adjust job descriptions, working conditions, and working hours — or develop whatever loopholes they found — as they have done in adapting to the Workers Compensation system.

It is understandable that American business is fighting universal health care rabidly. Every employer who has ever had even one employee file litigation for work injury knows what the company has at stake in universal health care. Under a universal health care system, employees and former employees will be able to get the medical reports upon which success of their litigation claims depend. There would become less stigmatization of physicians who write favorable reports for the injured rather than for the alleged injurer.

To understand the trends and the statistics, all one has to do is go to a public library, get an almanac off the reference shelves, and study the figures for who in the nation becomes disabled. The highest concentrations of disability are among the older minority members — the least powerful members of our culture. The tables of figures clearly show, however, that no group is entirely safe.

Health sciences tell us that if a person runs his or her body on caffeine and nicotine and sugar and fats instead of on green and varicolored vegetables, the body is going to break down. Less than six hours of sleep a night will cut 10 years off a person's life span. Sitting home and doing nothing does not result in contented disabled people; it results in higher medical bills followed by premature death. Active people who get balanced diets, sunshine, adequate rest, and who sleep well — live long lives.

Americans are an extremely productive people. Almost anyone can gauge the restless American activity rate. What one has to do is go out and around on any normal day of the year and then go out and around on Superbowl Sunday. There is a very profound difference in the hum of our society on a day when Americans stay home in their living rooms. Americans actually very rarely stay home in their living rooms — as comfortable as those may be as a rule.

If Americans in general really understood how the U.S.

personal injury litigation advocacy system functioned procedurally, they would form their own study groups, action groups, and lobbying groups to get the system corrected. The pubic doesn't know because the legal profession does know how very much it would have to change to adapt to a modern system.

This is a personal memoir of what happened to me and what I learned from it. I have the IQ and the academic training to be able to conduct the research interviews and to discern patterns within experience and to create meaning from such patterns, especially with the guidance of discussions with other specialized professionals. Certainly, the experience of others can vary. We have a large and complex nation, and the principle of States Rights is a real principle that does result in life experience varying from state to state. I have lived in six states, not all fifty.

You will perhaps have noticed that I have not quoted any laws to you. I am not an attorney and cannot do so. Non-attorneys can only discuss procedures, which is what I have done.

Not being a physician, I can only refer to what has worked personally for me. For what might work for you,

you must consult a licensed health professional for advice. Since I am not a medical doctor, the only advice I can give you is that you should seek immediate medical attention, if pain appears in your body, and keep seeking licensed medical help. Finding the right answers for yourself depends on continuing to ask, continuing to listen, and continuing to research.

Take your research findings back to your own physicians. Ask them for their evaluations of what you think you have figured out on your own or that your friends and family have told you. Your licensed medical team will either confirm your impressions or correct your misunderstandings. Then ask other physicians.

By interacting with physicians, you will discover for yourself which ones of your physicians stand up over the long haul, the ones who are in the medical profession because they love healing. Those are the ones in whose care you want to continue. They already know the score and have constructed their own practices for endurance in the face of adversity.

Health care professionals taught me how to survive. They can teach you how to, also. Many times, health care professionals sustain life by teaching self care.

About the Author

Herbert Anthem, Ph.D., instructed nursing and pre-med students in research methods on the university undergraduate level prior to sustaining an injury and through that injury learned about the contemporary health care system in ways not generally taught.

Professor Anthem's degrees are earned, academic ones, *not* medical ones. Tracing the currents in contemporary health care services has been a daily preoccupation for Dr. Anthem for over fifteen years.

Professor Anthem has written the present edition to increase general education. Nothing in this text should be construed as medical or legal advice. Medical and legal advice should be sought from licensed professionals in those professional fields.

herbertanthem@dr.com